Dedicated to new mothers

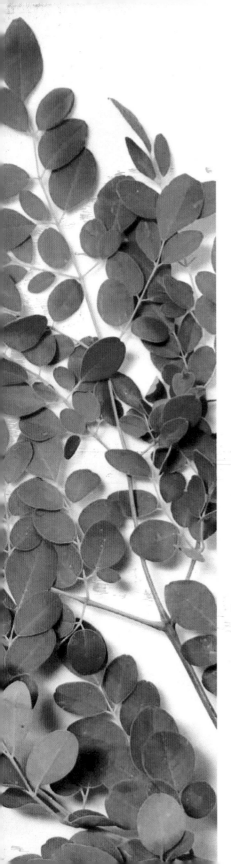

Editors: Khanh Hoa Nguyen, BA
Marilyn Wong, MD, MPH
frommotherstomothers@gmail.com

Disclaimer: This book is not intended as a substitute for the medical advice of physicians. The reader should consult a physician in matters relating to his/her health and particularly with respect to any symptoms that may require diagnosis or medical attention.

Printed by ASAP Quality Printing in Hayward, California

Available for sale at
Eastwind Books of Berkeley
2066 University Avenue
Berkeley, California 94704, USA.
Email: eastwindbooks@gmail.com
http://www.asiabookcenter.com

ISBN: 978-0-9963517-5-1

TABLE of CONTENTS

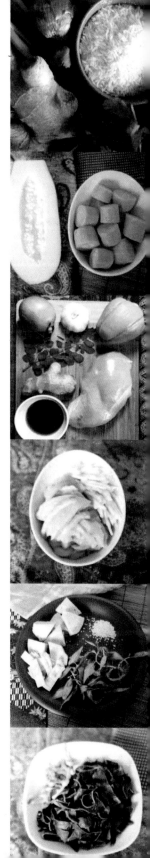

ABOUT US

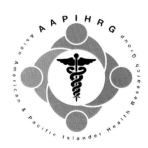

Asian American Pacific Islander Health Research Group (AAPIHRG) was organized in 2008 on the campus of the University of California at Berkeley by students and health professionals who were interested in promoting health in underserved immigrant and refugee communities. We fostered the research and the teaching of neglected health issues within these populations as part of an effort to educate and to prepare students to serve these communities in the future.

Each year, we recruited and trained a cohort of students to conduct research projects in the fall semester and to facilitate a lecture series in the spring semester that was partially based on the student's research topics.

In the fall of 2014, we began a project to collect and preserve information on traditional soups and dishes used in various AAPI cultures for the nourishment of new mothers during the month immediate after the birth of a child. This project was named the **Postpartum Nutrition Folklore Project**. The purpose was not to validate or invalidate the nutritional value of the recipes. Our aim was to collect and preserve information that would soon be lost.

Giving births and recovering from the birthing process are certainly not new phenomena. Women, through the ages, had to nourish themselves back to health as well as to ensure sufficient breast milk for the newborn during the postpartum period. Human survived and thrived because women not only learned how to care for themselves but also learned how to pass this knowledge to the next generation of mothers. Some of their wisdom was concentrated in the preparation of traditional postpartum soups and dishes.

Many AAPI immigrant women in the United States have been able to retain some knowledge on the postpartum nutritional belief of their ethnic culture through personal experience. However, within one generation, this traditional knowledge would often be lost due to the assimilation of the next generation into the mainstream Western culture.

Students from AAPI communities were in a unique position to inherit this traditional knowledge if they took an active part in seeking out the information from their mother, grandmother and relatives.

AAPIHRG, under the student leadership of Khanh Hoa Thi Nguyen, organized a group of students to collect postpartum recipes by interviewing their mothers, grandmothers and relatives. This book was a compilation of the collected recipes. The collection was a very small sample from a few Asian cultures. It would be our hope that this publication would encourage interest and research on a broader collection of recipes, on postpartum nutrition and, ultimately, on a scientific analysis of the nutritional value of these recipes.

A new group of students within AAPIHRG is already making plans to collect stories of multicultural postpartum practices and experiences. Much attention has been focused on postpartum depression in the United States in recent years. We intend to explore what should be and could be learned from women's experiences from around the world. Please support us in our efforts. We can be contacted at frommotherstomothers@gmail.com.

Marilyn P. Wong, MD, MPH
Co-Coordinator
Asian American Pacific Islander Health Research Group
UC Berkeley

FOREWORD

Eight years ago, when I gave birth to my first child, my mother flew from Los Angeles to New York to ensure that I would get what she considered to be the necessary post-partum diet to recover from childbirth and to re-establish a strong foundation for the rest of my life. Carrying two suitcases, one full of her own belongings and another filled with medicinal herbs and frozen but freshly killed chickens, she took control of the kitchen and prepared Cantonese postpartum meals that would help heal and strengthen my body. Among the many items she cooked for me, my most treasured dish is the quintessential Cantonese postpartum concoction of ginger, sweetened vinegar, pig trotters, and whole chicken eggs. I remember well from my childhood days this distinctly body-warming, sweet and sour concoction with a deep brown color and rich sinuous texture. As a child, I looked forward to every opportunity when I can visit families with newborns just so I can drink this special soup reserved for these occasions. In my own postpartum recovery, I took pleasure in every gulp, savoring the complexly rich flavors and the equally intense fragrance it produced. The concoction induced heat that radiated from my core and provided extraordinary warmth. It nourished not just the body but also the soul and senses as well.

There are few transformative events that mark one's passage through life and spark significant changes in one's emotional, cultural, and physiological states. Without doubt, giving birth ranks as one of the most important life-changing events in women's lives. Among most Asian cultures, childbirth animates elaborate sets of food practices, bodily regimens, and rituals that reveal established beliefs of food, nutrition, the body, and women's postpartum health.

In Chinese culture—and Asian cultures, more generally— food is often treated like medicine, in the sense that each food item is assessed for its medicinal or health value and known for its particular effects on the body (i.e. warming or cooling, drying or moisture-inducing). The idea is that by controlling and adjusting everyday food intake (the items, the amounts, and the combinations), one can recalibrate one's health according to the changing needs of the body. Food consumption, then, serves to regulate health, treat ailments, and prevent imbalances that can lead to illness. By becoming aware of the effects of food and sharpening attunement to one's bodily changes, one can make conscious decisions on food consumption to aid in positive nourishment and healing. Given this relationship to food and the life-changing event of childbirth, many Asian cultures are endowed with abundant recipes and bodily regimens associated with postpartum recovery. These recipes, beliefs, and practices form an important part of women's knowledge that is passed from one generation to the next or laterally among women of the same generation through oral narratives, observation, and the act of cooking together.

In the context of migration and becoming a minoritized group, Asian migrants face a number of factors that make it difficult to sustain culturally distinct practices and beliefs. These factors include the weakening of inter-generational communication through loss of native languages, the lack of access to specific food items, and the loss of value placed on culturally specific knowledge. Nonetheless, even in the context of these challenges, ethnic Asians in the United States and elsewhere in diaspora continue to find these postpartum practices and beliefs culturally significant and personally meaningful. Asian mothers and grandmoth ers continue to prepare their special recipes that help replenish and rebalance postpartum bodies, as well as induce breast milk production to nourish growing infants. In fact, when women relatives are not available to do so, young Asian mothers can now purchase month-long postpartum meals from local chefs who specialize in this culinary tradition. Far from disappearing, Asian women of various ethnic backgrounds continue to embrace, believe, and consume these culturally prescribed postpartum diets.

This volume is a testament of the AAPI Health Research Group's commitment to documenting and preserving the centuries-old recipes and practices of postpartum food preparation. The students collected recipes from women of various ethnic Asian backgrounds—Vietnamese, Cambodian, Hmong, Filipino, Korean, and Chinese— and published them in both English and their respective native languages. As a whole, the volume helps preserve AAPI women's knowledge, reclaims their ability to care and nourish their own bodies, and promotes cultural and culinary empowerment. By writing each recipe in both English and its respective Asian language, the book gives access to a much broader audience and facilitates conversation across generations, linguistic abilities, and geography. English, Vietnamese, Cambodian, Hmong, Filipino, Korean, and Chinese language readers can all delight in recreating these recipes and benefitting from this collective knowledge.

Thanks to this group of dedicated students and their maverick mentor Marilyn Wong, M.D., we finally have the first edition of postpartum recipes from various Asian ethnic groups in the United States. It is the first of its kind, and they should be proud of their accomplishment in not only safe-guarding AAPI women's cultural knowledge of health and nutrition but also giving all of us access to these time-tested recipes for women's postpartum health!

Lok Siu, Ph.D.
Associate Professor
Asian American and Asian Diaspora Studies Program
Ethnic Studies Department
UC Berkeley

Message from the project coordinator

I'm so thrilled to introduce our postpartum recipe book to you. Over the last two years, our members have worked very hard on every single aspect of this book, from interviewing our relatives for postpartum recipes to cooking and taking pictures of the dishes. We've collected over 30 recipes from 6 different cultures. The recipes presented in this book are the ones that you can easily find the ingredients in your local markets. Most of us are college students with little cooking experience. We cooked and tasted these dishes and soups ourselves. Much to our surprise, the dishes were rather simple to cook and came out delicious. I believe any beginner chef or mother who is cooking our postpartum recipes for the first time will do just fine. I also hope that you will enjoy the cooking and tasting these postpartum dishes.

Our project is entirely student-run, so your support means a lot to us. Your purchase of this book will help us print more copies and continue to share our culture's traditional postpartum knowledge. Here, I want to thank my members for their precious time and beautiful work. I also want to thank Dr. Marilyn Wong, Momo Chang, professional chef Bryant Terry, and UC Berkeley Professors Lok Siu and Harvey Dong for their time and many good advice.

Khanh-Hoa Thi Nguyen
B.A. Public Health and Molecular & Cellular Biology
UC Berkeley

VIETNAMESE

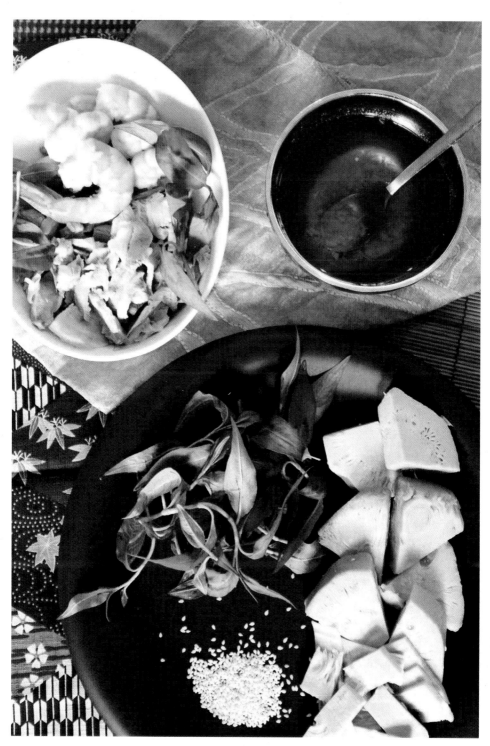

Canh đu đủ hầm giò heo

2 pound đu đủ non xanh

2 giò heo đã được cắt ra khúc nhỏ dày 3-4 cm

1 muỗng nước nắm

1 muỗng muối

½ muỗng tiêu

½ muỗng đường

hành lá

ngò (tuỳ ý)

1. Rửa sạch chân heo với nước lạnh, rồi cho vào nồi nước lớn.

2. Hầm trong vòng 1-2 tiếng cho đến khi giò heo mềm.

3. Thường xuyên vớt bọt.

4. Trong khi chờ đợi, rửa và gọt vỏ đu đủ. Bỏ hết hạt bên trong, rồi cắt đu đủ thành từng khúc dày khoảng 2 cm.

5. Khi thấy giò heo đã mềm, cho vào đu đủ và nấu đến khi đu đủ mềm.

6. Tắt bếp, cho vào nước nắm, muối, tiêu, đường. Cho thêm hành ngò đã được thái nhỏ vào.

Papaya Soup with Slow-cooked Pig Feet

2 pounds of green papaya

2 pig feet that have been cut into small pieces of 3-4 cm thick

1 tablespoon of fish sauce

1 tablespoon of salt

½ teaspoon of black pepper

½ teaspoon of sugar

julienned spring onion

cilantro (optional)

1. Thoroughly wash the pig feet in cold water, and then place them in a big pot filled with water.

2. Cook for 1-2 hours until the pig feet become soft.

3. Constantly remove the impurities floating on top of the pot.

4. While waiting, wash the papaya and peel its skin. Remove the seeds and cut the papaya into small pieces of 2 cm thick.

5. Once the pig feet become soft, add papaya pieces and cook until they become soft.

6. Turn off heat, add fish sauce, salt, black pepper, and sugar. Add some julienned spring onion and cilantro.

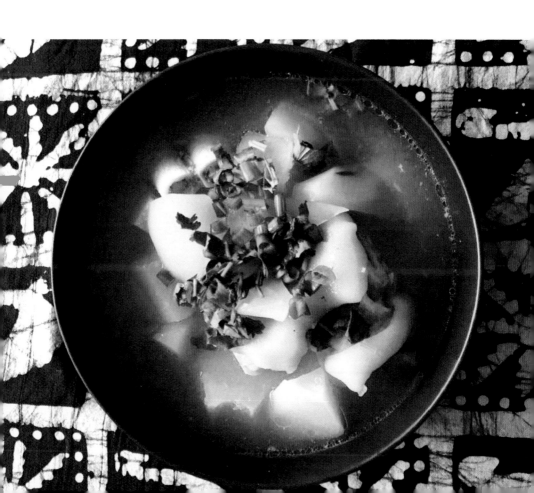

Giá Xào Tôm

1 pound giá

100 gram (¼ lb) tôm

1 củ hành thái lát

2 muỗng nước mắm

½ muỗng đường

chút tiêu

hành

ngò

1. Tôm bóc vỏ, loại đường chỉ đen trên lưng, rửa sạch.

2. Ướp với 1 muỗng cà phê nước nắm.

3. Bắc bếp, cho ít dầu ăn vào chảo rồi cho hành củ đã thái vào chảo.

4. Khi thấy hành đã thơm (20-30 giây), cho tôm vào chảo và nấu đến khi chín.

5. Cho giá vào xào chung cho đến khi giá chín (khoảng 10-15 phút).

6. Tắt bếp. Cho 1 muỗng nước nắm và nửa muỗng đường vào. Rải chút tiêu và cho thêm hành ngò thái nhuyễn.

Bean Sprouts with Shrimps

1 pound of bean sprouts

100 grams (¼ lb) shrimps

1 whole thinly sliced shallot

2 tablespoons of fish sauce

½ tablespoon of sugar

a pinch of black pepper

spring onion

cilantro

1. Rinse and deshell shrimps, then place them in a bowl.

2. Add a tablespoon of fish sauce to the bowl.

3. Place your pan on medium heat, and then add oil and sliced shallots.

4. Once shallots turn light brown (after 20-30 seconds), add shrimps.

5. Add bean sprouts and stir for about 10-15 minutes.

6. Turn off heat. Add 1 tablespoon of fish sauce and half a tablespoon of sugar. Sprinkle a bit of black pepper and add chopped spring onion and cilantro on top.

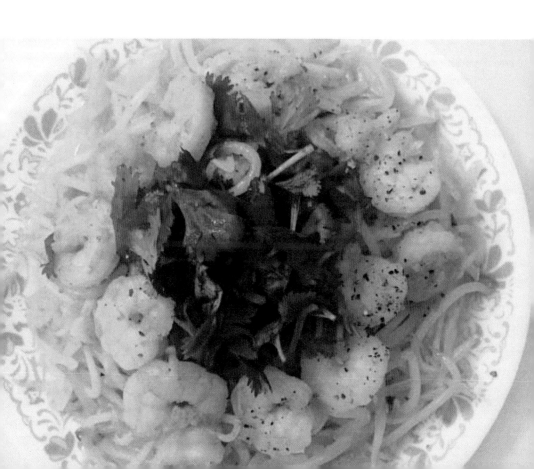

Gỏi Mít Non

*1 quả mít non
hoặc 2 lon mít non*

1 muỗng canh nước mắm tỏi

thịt heo và/hoặc tôm luộc

30 gram mè

vài nhánh rau răm

1. Luộc mít cho mềm (khoảng 30 phút), rồi vớt ra thái mỏng.

2. Rang mè trên chảo. Cho vào một cái tô và giã nhỏ.

3. Trong một tô lớn, trộn mít, mè, thịt luộc và/hoặc tôm luộc, nước nắm tỏi, rau răm rồi trộn đều trong khoảng 10-15 phút.

4. Xếp ra đĩa và cho thêm mè lên trên.

Young Jackfruit Salad

1 whole young jackfruit or 2 cans of young jackfruit

1 ladle of fish sauce vinaigrette

boiled pork and/or shrimps

30 grams of sesame seeds

Vietnamese mint

1. Boil pieces of jackfruit until they become soft (usually takes about 30 minutes). Then take them out and slice them thinly.

2. Pan roast sesame seeds. Then place in a bowl and lightly grind.

3. In a salad bowl, add sliced jackfruit, sesame seeds, cooked pork and/or shrimps, fish sauce vinaigrette, chopped Vietnamese mint leaves and mix everything for about 10-15 minutes.

4. Plate your salad and sprinkle some sesame seeds on top.

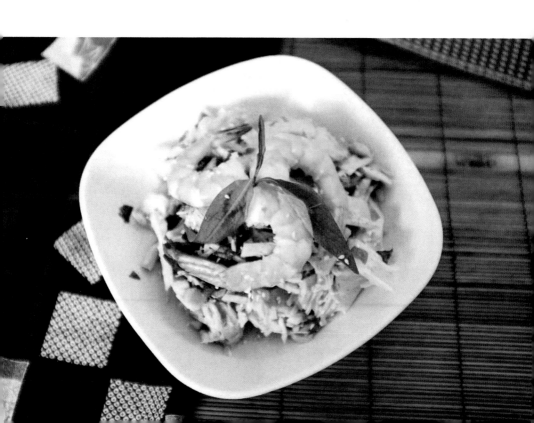

CAMBODIAN

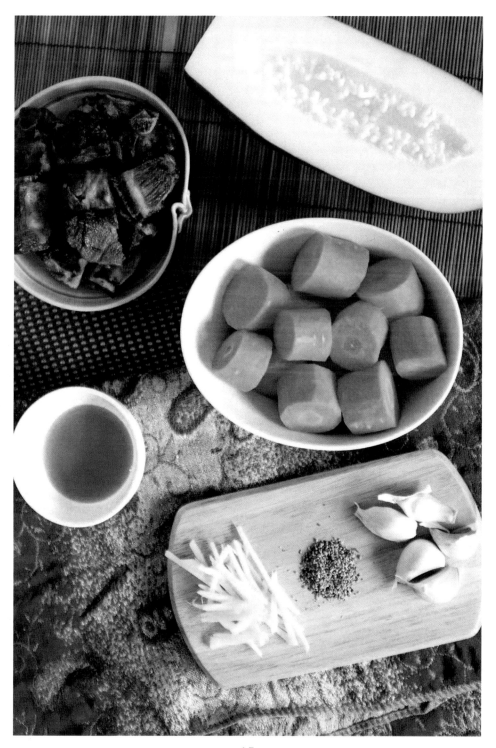

ឆាខ្ទឹសាច់មាន់

ទ្រូងមាន់២ដុំ ហាន់ជាដុំតូចៗ
ខ្ទឹមបារាំង១ ហាន់ជាកង់តូចៗ
ខ្ទឹហាន់រួច 1.5ពែង
ខ្ទឹមស ចំនួន៣កំពីស
ចិញ្ច្រាំ អោយល្អិត
ទឹកត្រី ២ស្លាបព្រាបាយ
ប៉ូរចេង ១ស្លាបព្រាការហ្វេ
ស្ករ ១ស្លាបព្រាការហ្វេ
ប្រេងឆា ២ស្លាបព្រាបាយ

1. ច្របល់ ទឹកត្រី oyster sauce/ប្រេងខ្លង ប៉ូរចេង ស្ករ រួចច្របល់ជាមួយសាច់មាន់

2. ដាក់ខ្ទះអោយក្ដៅ ដាក់ប្រេងឆា ខ្ទឹម និង ខ្ទី

3. បើកភ្លើង អោយខ្លាំង រួចឆារហូតដល់ខ្ទីទន់

4. ដាក់សាច់មាន់ចូល

5. ពេលមាន់ឆ្អិន ដាក់ខ្ទឹមបារាំង រួចចំអិនរហូតដល់ខ្ទឹមបារាំងទន់

Ginger Sauteed Chicken

2 chicken breasts, cut into strips

1 onion, cut into strips

1.5 cups of julienned ginger

3 cloves of minced garlic

2 tablespoons of fish sauce

1 teaspoon of sugar

2 tablespoons of cooking oil

1. Combine fish sauce, oyster sauce, and sugar. Mix together with chicken.

2. In a hot pan, add oil, garlic and ginger.

3. Sauté until ginger is soft.

4. Add chicken to pan.

5. When chicken is cooked, add onion and cook with lid on until onion is tender.

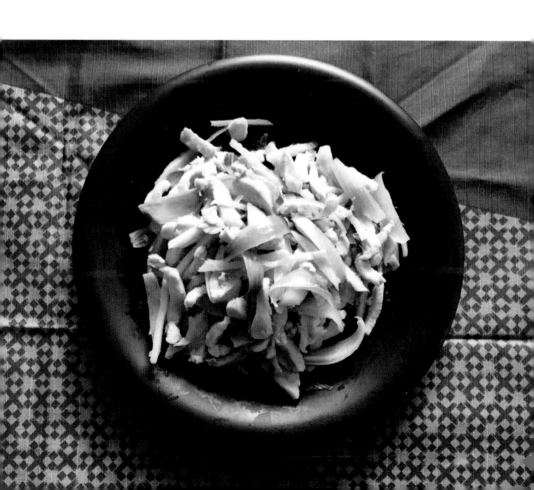

ខសាច់ជ្រក

សាច់ជ្រកពីរ៣ធាន ២ធាន កាត់ជាដុំបួនជ្រុងប្រវែង ១អិញ ខ្លី១ពែង ហាន់ក្រាស់១ ខ្លីមស ២ដុំ បកសំបករួច ម្រេច ១ស្លាបព្រាបាយ អំបិល ១ស្លាបព្រាបាយ សូរ ៣ស្លាបព្រាបាយ ប៉ីចេង ១ស្លាបព្រាការហ្ម ទឹកត្រី ២ ទឹកសុីអ៊ីវខ្មៅ១ស្លាបព្រាបាយ ទឹកពាពែង

1. ដាក់អំបិល ម្រេច ខ្លីមសចូលក្នុងត្បាល់ រួចបុកបញ្ចូលគ្នា
2. ដាក់ទឹកត្រី សូរ ប៉ីចេង រួចច្របាច់ជាមួយសាច់ជ្រក
3. ដាក់ខ្លីចូល
4. កំលោចសូរ រួចច្របល់ជាមួយសាច់ជ្រក ក្នុងឆ្នាំងជំ
5. ដាក់ទឹកពាពែង រួចគ្របគំរបឆ្នាំង ចំអិនរយៈពេល៤៥នាទីដោយប្រើភ្លើ ងល្មម

18

Braised and Caramelized Pork Stew

*2 pounds of pork belly,
cut into 1 inch cubes*

1 cup ginger, sliced thick

2 heads garlic, peeled

1 tablespoon of black pepper

1 tablespoon of salt

3 tablespoon of sugar

*2 tablespoons of fish sauce or
dark soy sauce*

3 cups of water

1. In a mortar and pestle, combine salt, black pepper, garlic and pound into a paste.

2. In a bowl, message the pork with the paste, fish sauce, and sugar.

3. Add the ginger.

4. Caramelize the pork mixture in a large pot.

5. Add 3 cups of water, cover and braise the pork on medium heat for 45 minutes.

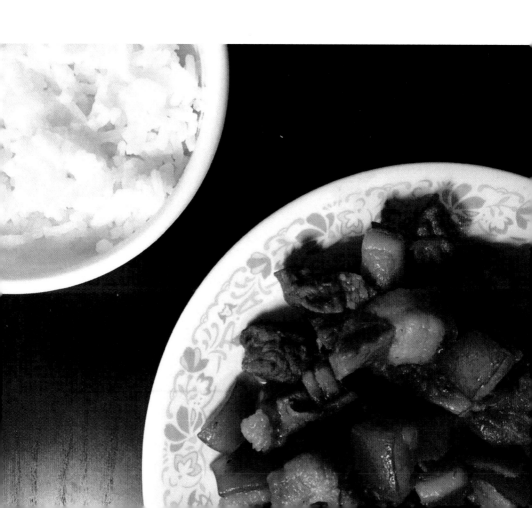

បបរមាន់ឈាមជ្រូក

ទ្រូងមាន់ ២
ថ្លើងទ្រូងមាន់ ២
ឈាមជ្រូក ១ជោន
ស៊ុបមាន់ ៦ពែង
ខ្ទិៈពែង ហាន់ក្រាស់ៗ
ខ្ទឹម ៦កំពីស
អង្ករ ១ពែង
នៃពៅ 1/4ពែង
ទឹកត្រី ២ស្លាបព្រាបាយ
ម្រេច ១ស្លាបព្រាបាយ
អំបិល ១ស្លាបព្រាការហ្វេ
ស្ពឹកខ្ទឹម ១គុម្ព ហាន់ល្អិតៗ
cilantro/ជីវ៉ាន់ស៊ុយ ១គុម្ព
ចិញ្ច្រាំអោយល្អិត

របៀបធ្វើនឈាមជ្រូក
1. ដាំទឹក ១ឆ្នាំង
2. ដាក់ឈាមជ្រូកចូលទាំងអស់ ដាក់ស្ងោររយៈពេល ២០នាទី ប្រើភ្លើងតិចៗ
3. លើកចេញ ទុកអោយត្រជាក់ រួចកាត់ជាដុំបួនជ្រុងប្រវែង១អិញ

របៀបធ្វើនបបរ
1. ចាក់ទឹកស៊ុបមាន់ និងទឹក៦ពែង ចូលក្នុងឆ្នាំងដំមួយ រួចទុកអោយពុះ
2. ដាក់ ខ្ទឹម ខ្ទី ផៃពៅ ម្រេច និង សាច់មាន់

Rice Porridge with Pig Blood Curd and Chicken

2 chicken breasts

2 chicken breast carcass (bones)

1 pound coagulated pig blood curd

6 cups chicken broth (home made or store bought)

1 cup ginger, sliced thick

6 cloves garlic

1 cup of raw rice

¼ cup fermented daikon radish

2 tablespoons of fish sauce

1 tablespoons of black pepper

1 teaspoon of salt

1 bunch green onion, thinly sliced

1 bunch cilantro, minced

TO PREPARE PIG BLOOD CURD

1. Boil a pot of water.

2. Add entire block of pig blood curd into the water and simmer on low heat, covered, for 20 minutes.

3. Remove from water and let it cool. Cut pig blood curd into 1 inch cubes, set aside.

TO PREPARE PORRIDGE

1. In a large pot, add chicken broth, 6 cups of water and bring to a rolling boil.

2. Add garlic, ginger, fermented daikon radish, black pepper, sliced chicken and prepared pig blood curd.

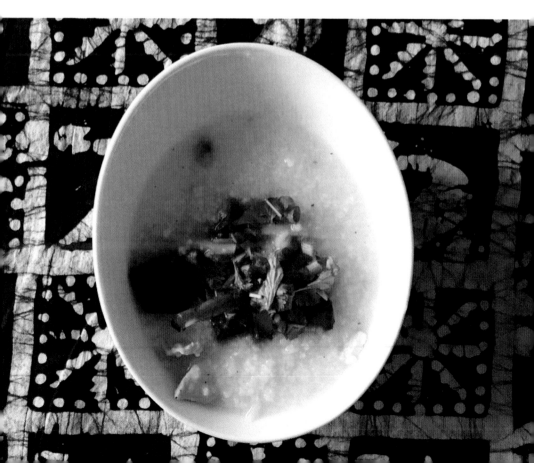

ឆ្លើងស៊ុបជាមួយសាច់គោ
ការ៉ុតនិងផ្លែល្ហុងខ្ចី

ឆ្លើងសាច់គោចំនួន៥ជោន ការ៉ុត១ជោន,ចិតសំបកចេញនិងកាត់ទៅជាកំណាត់ 1,5 អ៊ីញ ផ្លែល្ហុងខ្ចី ចិតសំបកចេញហើយកាត់ទៅជាកំណាត់ 1,5 អ៊ីញ ខ្ញីហាន់រួច(ហាន់ជាថិនិតគូឡេម)ខ្ញីមស 5 កំពីស ទឹកគ្រឿងអោន ម្រេចខ្ទៀ១ស្លាបព្រាការហ្វេ អំបិល១ស្លាបព្រាការហ្វេ ទឹក 16 តែង (1 ហ្គាឡុន)

1. ដាំទឹកជាមួយឆ្អឹងផ្តុំអោយពុះ។
2. ដាក់ឆ្អឹងគោ, ខ្ញី, ខ្ទឹម, ទឹកត្រី, ម្រេចខ្ទៀនិងអំបិល។
3. ស្ងោររយៈពេល5នាទី រួចហើយបន្ថយភ្លើង ប្រើភ្លើងតិចៗគ្របគំរបឆ្នាំងហើយម្សាស់រយៈពេល2ម៉ោង។ បើកគំរបឆ្នាំងរួចដួសពុះខ្លាញ់ចេញ។
4. បន្ថែមល្ហុងនិងការ៉ុត។
5.ចំអិនដោយប្រើភ្លើងល្មមរហូតដល់បន្លែទុំ យ។ លែ/ដាក់គ្រឿងតម្រូវតាមចំណង់រសជាតិ។

Beef Bone Soup with Carrots and Young Papaya

5 pounds of beef bones

1 pound of carrots, peeled and cut into 1.5 inch chunks

1 pound of young papaya, peeled and cut into 1.5 inch chunks

¼ cup of sliced ginger

5 cloves garlic

1 ounce of fish sauce

1 tablespoon of black pepper

1 teaspoon of salt

16 cups water (1 gallon)

1. In a large pot, bring water to a rolling boil.

2. Add beef bones, ginger, garlic, fish sauce, black pepper and salt.

3. Keep it at a rolling boil for 5 minutes then turn the heat to the lowest setting, cover and let simmer for 2 hours. Skim the fat off the soup.

4. Add papaya and carrots.

5. Cook on medium heat until veggies are tender. Adjust seasoning to taste.

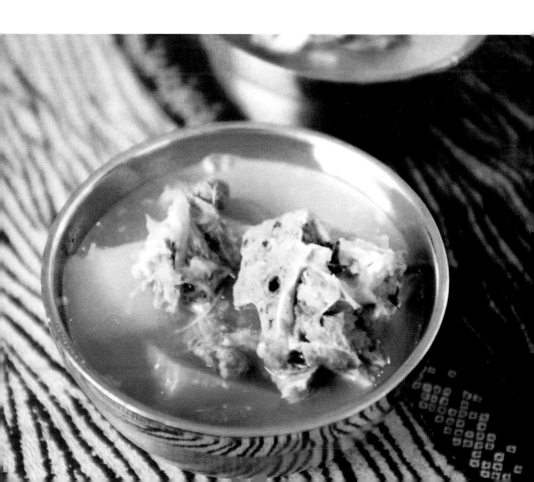

H'MONG

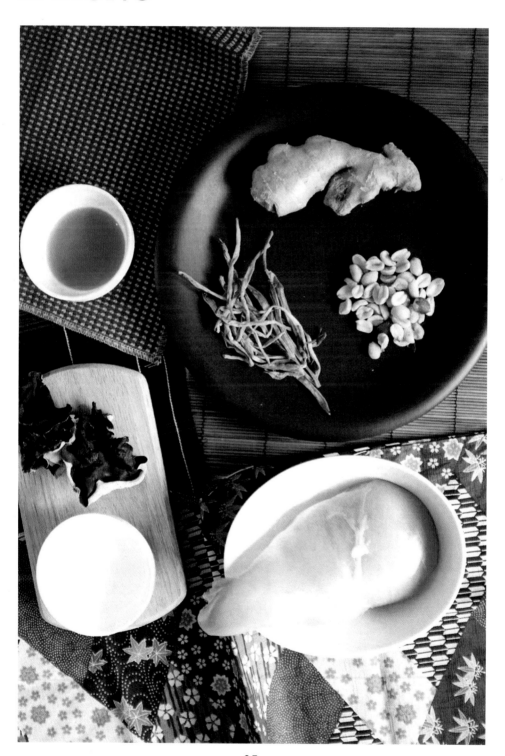

Qaib Hau Nrog Tshuaj

1 tug qaib yug tom teb

10-14 khob dej

1 tug tauj dub

Cov Tshuaj tseem ceeb: Muab thaj tsam li ntawm 2-3 khob tshuaj hau nrog tus qaib. 2-3 khob no muaj tag nrho cov tshuaj uas hais raws li tom qab no:

Tshuaj qab lo

Zej Ntshua Ntuag

Xsuv Ntsim

Kuab Nplias Dib

Pawj qaib

Tseej ntug

1. Hau dej hauv lauj kaub.

2. Muaj ib rab riam loj los tsoo tauj dub, ces muaj tso hauv lub lauj kaub. Ua li no thiaj tsw qab.

3. Yaug thiab hlais tus qaib muab ua 12-16 daim nqaij, nyob ntawm qhov koj n3yiam loj los me. Yog hau raws li Hmoob ib txwm hau qaib los, daim tawv, lub caj dab, thiab ob tus kos taw ntawm tus qaib yuav tsum hau nrog tib si.

4. Thaum dej npau, muab nqaij qaib tso rau.

Boiled Chicken with Special Herbs

1 cage-free, farm-raised chicken

10-14 cups of water

1 stalk of lemongrass

Special Herbs: Several sprigs of each herb will be used in the soup for a total of 2-3 cups of loosely packed herbs. *

Angelica

Zej Ntshua Ntuag

Xsuv Ntsim

Kuab Nplias Dib

Pawj qaib (sweet flag)

Tseej ntug (common dayflower)

1. Boil water in a stockpot.

2. Smash the stalk of lemongrass with a cooking pounder or a heavy knife, and add it to the pot. The smashing will release the aroma of the lemongrass to the soup.

3. Rinse and cut the chicken into 12-16 pieces, depending on how you like the size. For a traditional soup, the skin is left on as well as the head and feet.

4. Once water is boiling, add chicken and cook until done.

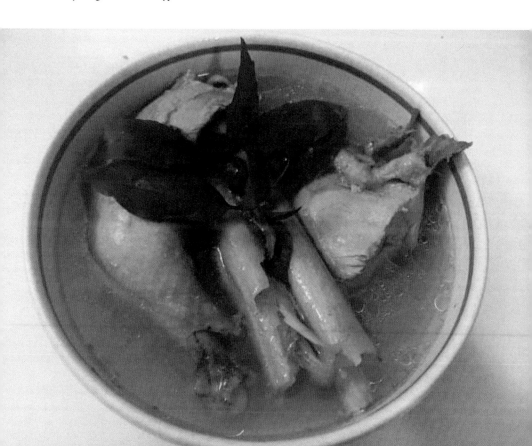

Qaib Hau Nrog Qhiav Thiab Cawv

500 grams ntawm cov hauv siab qaib

200 grams ntawm cov qhiav

100 mL cawv

1 tes daylily

1 tes nceb ntswm

50 grams ntawm cov txiv laum faj xeeb

3 dia ntawm cov sesame roj

½ teaspoon ntawm cov ntsev

(muaj qij thiab sesame roj los tau)

1. Tsau daylily thiab nceb ntswm ib hmo nkaus. Muaj tsi dej thiab ntxuav kom huv.

2. Hlais tus qaib lub hauv siab ua ib daim ib daim ib cm tuab.

3. Siv ib lub yias loj ces muab sesame roj nchuav rau hauv thiab siv hluav taws kom siab. Ces muaj ob peb nplais qhiav ntxiv rau hauv lub yias kom muaj 2 feeb kom tsw qab.

4. Ntxiv nqaij qaib thiab do kom muaj ob feeb kom nws pib daj. Ces tov cawv rau, yog tsis muaj dej txaus ua kom npau ces ntxiv dej rau. Ces cia nws npau kom muaj 5 feeb.

5. Ntxiv daylily thiab nceb ntswm

6. Cia nws npau kom muaj thaj tsam li 50 feeb.

Chicken Soup with Ginger and Wine

500 grams of chicken breast

200 grams of julienned ginger

100 mL white rice wine

1 handful of daylily

1 handful of black fungus

50 grams of peanuts

3 tablespoons of sesame oil

½ teaspoon of salt

(optional garlic and sesame oil)

1. Soak daylily and black fungus overnight. Drain water and rinse clean.

2. Chop chicken breast into 1cm thick slices.

3. In a large wok or pan, heat sesame oil over high heat. Add ginger slices and cook for 2 minutes until fragrant.

4. Add chicken and cook for 2 minutes until slightly browned. Add white rice wine (water if needed), and bring to boil. Then cook for 5 minutes.

5. Add daylily and black fungus.

6. Leave it to boil for about 50 minutes.

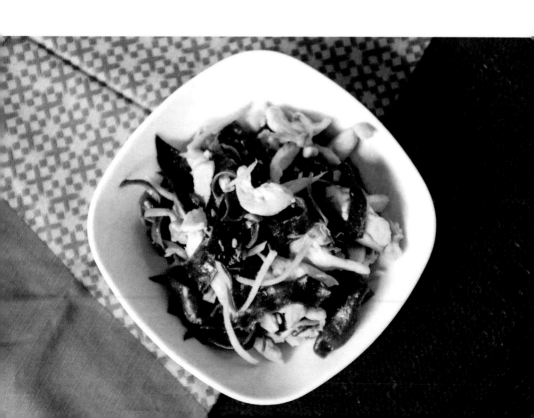

FILIPINO

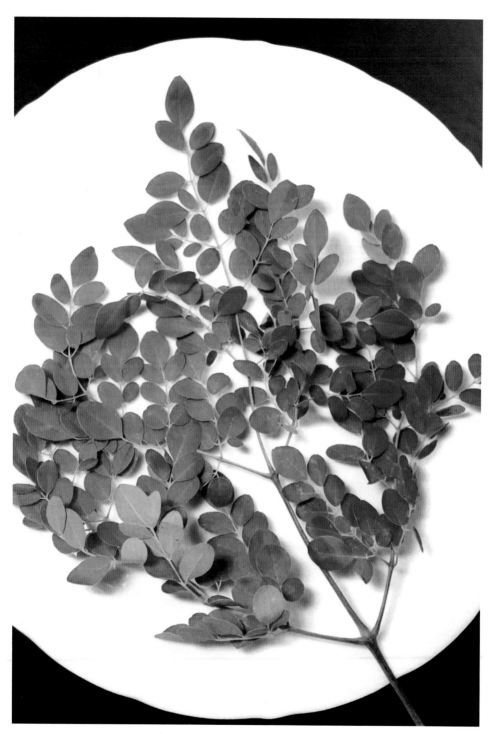

Tinola

tatlo o apat cloves ng bawang

isang maliit na sibuyas

isang inch ng luya

anong parte ng chicken

tubig

asin

paminta

sayote

malunggay

patis

ginisa mix

1. Kuskusin ng asin ang manok para maalis ang lansa at dulas nito. Ang procesa na ito ay magbibigay ng malinis at walang lansa sa paglasa. 2. Banlawan ang manok sa tubig hanggang maalis ang dugo nito. Alisin ang mga dahon ng malunggay sa stem.

2. Igisa ang mga bawang, sibuyas, at luya sa konti langgis.

3. Idagdag ang manok na may konting paminta at asin.

4. Hintayin hanggan kayumanggi ang kulay ng manok.

5. Lagyan ng tubig ang kaserola para sa sabaw. Hintayin hanggang maluto na maige ang manko at kumulo ang tubig.

6. Alisin ang mga bumubula sa ibabaw kumukulong tubig.

7. Lagyan ng sayote ang kumukulong tubig at hintayan hanggang ito ay maluto.

8. Idagdag ang patis at ginisa mix sa putahe hanggang sanghayon sa inyong maglasa. Mag ingat na hindi masyado mapaalat ang sabaw ng tinola.

9. Idagdag na ang malunggay. Maghintay ng dalawang minutos at ipatay ang kalan. Kaunting minutos lang ang kailangan para maluto ang malunggay.

Tinola

chicken (any part, i.e. 1 chicken breast)

sayote (chayote)

malunggay (moringga)

3-4 cloves of garlic

1 small onion

1 inch of ginger

water

salt

black pepper

patis (fish sauce)

ginisa mix

1. Rub salt on the chicken in order to remove its slime for a cleaner, fresher aftertaste. Rinse until all blood is gone.

2. Detach moringga leaves from stem, and set them aside.

3. Sauté 3-4 cloves of diced garlic, one small diced onion, and 1 inch diced ginger with little oil.

4. Add chicken (can be legs, wings, etc) with a dash of grated black pepper. Wait until chicken turns brown.

5. Add water for the soup. Wait until chicken is fully cook and bring it to a boil. Remove the foam that builds up while boiling.

6. Add sayote and wait until cooked.

7. Add fish sauce and ginisa mix to your liking. Careful to not make it too salty!

8. Add moringga leaves. Wait for 2 minutes or so and turn off heat. It only takes a couple of seconds for the leaves to cook.

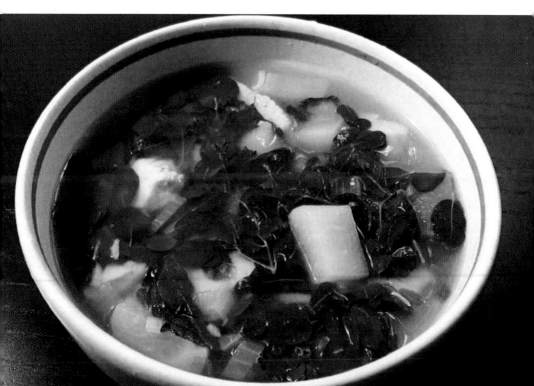

Tulia

tulia

patis

Nor seasoning

kamatis

at luya

kung gusto na may gulay

pwedeng idagdag ang patola

1. Hugasan ang mga tulia ng tubig.

2. Lagyan ng tubig ang kaserola kasama ang kamatis at luya na nakahiwa ng maliliit na peraso. Ipakulo ang tubig.

3. Kapag kumukulo na ang tubig, lagyan ito ng patis, Nor seasoning, at ang mga tulia. Kung iluluto na may kasamang gulay, idagdag rin ang patola.

4. Kapag bumuka na ang mga tulia, luto na ito.

Tulia

tulia (Manila clams)

patis (fish sauce)

Nor seasoning

Optional:

patola

tomato

ginger

1. Rinse the tulia.

2. Add water into a pan with diced tomato and ginger. Bring to boil.

3. Once boiling, add patis and Nor seasoning (if you would like vegetables, add patola).

4. Add tulia and cook until the tulia opens.

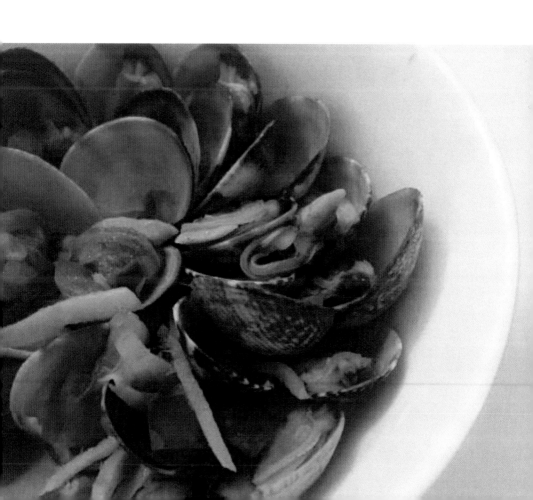

KOREAN

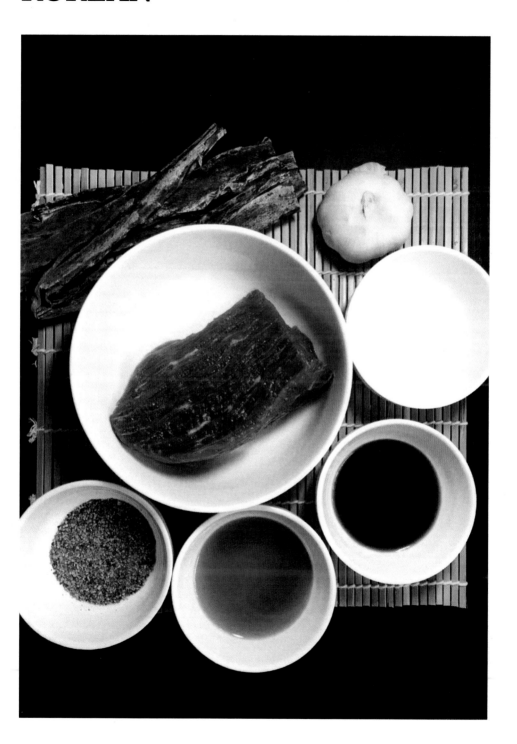

소고기 미역국

미역: 100g
소고기: ½ lb
소금: 2 tsp
간장: 3 tbs
후츄: ½ tsp
마늘: 2 tbs
물: 1.5 L
참기름: 1 tbs

1. 미역을 물의 1시간정도 불린다

2. 소고기를 납작 납작하게 썰어 놓는다

3. 냄비에 불을 켜서 소고기를 넣고 참기름을1
스푼 넣어 볶는다

4. 고기가 익으면 불려서 씻은 미역을
3번에 넣어서 같이 5분정도 간장과소금을 적당
히 넣어 볶는다

5. 다음은4번에 물을 넣어서 끓기
시작하면 마늘을 넣고 간을 맞춰 20분 정도 끓
은후에 불을 끈다

Seaweed Soup with Beef

100 grams of seaweed

2 teaspoon of salt

½ pound beef

3 teaspoon of soy sauce

½ teaspoon of black pepper

2 teaspoon of (minced) garlic

1.5 liters of water

1 tablespoon of sesame oil

1. Soak dried seaweed in water for at least 1 hour.

2. Slice the beef into thin slices.

3. Place a pot over the stove and add sesame oil and beef.

4. As the beef cooks, place the seaweed in the pot as well. Add the soy sauce, salt, and pepper. Pan fry for 5 minutes.

5. Add water. Once it boils, add garlic and add more salt, soy sauce, or pepper to match your taste.

6. Stew for at least 20 minutes before serving.

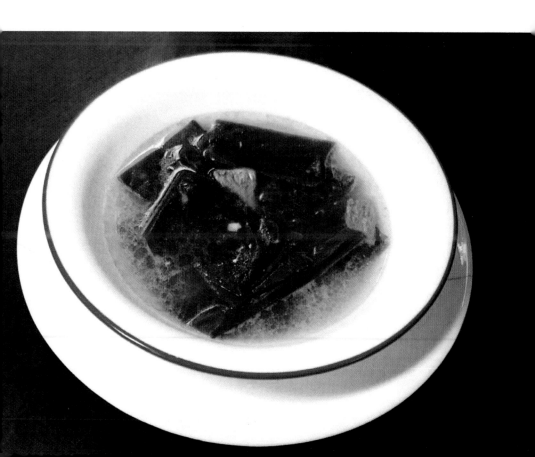

CHINESE

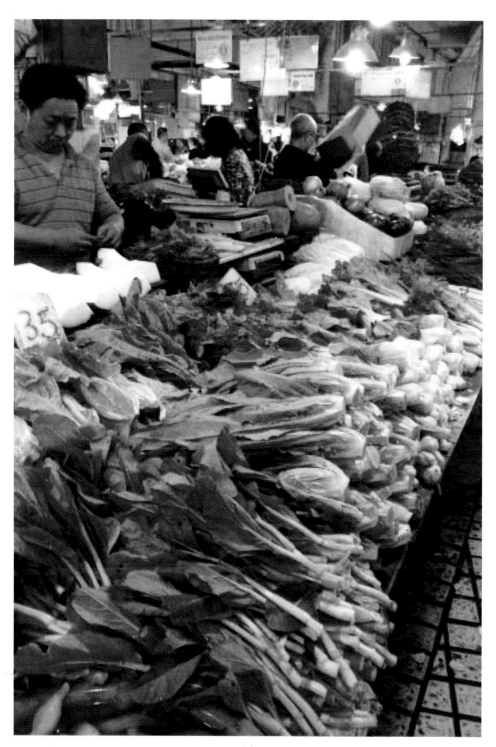

麻油腰只

腰只2份

薑(切片)15公克

枸杞5公克

水600cc

麻油2茶匙

雞粉0.5茶匙

米酒100cc

醬油3大匙

砂糖1.5茶匙

太白粉5大匙

胡椒少許

1. 將豬腎臟洗淨，並切除豬腎背後的血管和組織，煮的時候才不會有腥味。

2. 用刀子輕輕在豬腎表面畫上幾刀，在烹煮時才能吸收調味。將豬腎以三大匙的醬油、一點五匙的糖、五大匙的太白粉、以及些許胡椒粉醃製。醃製，並冰在冰箱幾小時到一天。

3. 醃製完成後，表面會呈現漂亮的醬油色。將豬腎在沸水中川燙，洗去多餘血水與過多的調味，再泡浸至冰水中。此步驟可以讓腰只在烹煮後口感更加清脆。

4. 以中火烹煮，在平底鍋上加入少許油，油熱之後加入薑片爆香。約過30秒至1分鐘、完全爆香之後，轉成小火並加入豬腎，稍微拌炒一下。

5. 當豬腎約百分之80煮熟時，加入米酒、水、麻油。依然稍微做拌炒即可，等至鍋裡水沸騰及米酒蒸發。

6. 關火，先加三至五滴麻油至要盛放的盤子裡，同時可加點雞精，最後將鍋裡的豬腎放進盤子，即完成。

Pig Kidneys in Sesame Oil

2 kidneys

15 grams of ginger

5 grams of chinese wolfberry

600 mL water

2 teaspoons of sesame oil

½ teaspoon chicken essence

100mL cooking wine

3 tablespoons of soy sauce

1.5 teaspoons of sugar

5 tablespoons of potato starch

some pepper

1. Score the kidney with a knife to increase the surface area for better flavor absorption.

2. Place kidneys into a bowl with 3 table-spoons of soy sauce, 1.5 teaspoons of sugar, 5 tablespoon of potato starch, and some pepper. Then, refrigerate for a few hours to one day to let marinade.

3. When the kidneys are sufficiently marinaded, they will have a good aroma and soy sauce-colored appearance. Then, blanch the kidneys in hot water to wash away the additional salty flavor. Followed by soaking in iced water. This step will make the kidneys more crispy after cooking.

4. Heat pan at medium heat. Add oil. When the pan is hot, add ginger and stir fry it. When the smell of ginger becomes stronger, which may take about 30 seconds to 1 minute, turn heat on low and add kidneys to the pan. Stir once in a while.

5. When the kidneys are about 80% done, add the cooking wine first, and then add the water and Chinese wolfberry (goji berry). Stir once in a while until the water boils and wine evapo-rates.

6. Turn off heat, and add 3-5 drops of sesame oil. To serve, put some chicken essence on a plate and add the kidneys.

月子姜炒飯

1碗 剩米飯
2個 雞蛋
1大塊 姜
適量 鹽

1. 姜去皮（不去皮效果更好)
2. 將姜剁成碎
3. 鍋內放油燒熱
4. 放入姜碎沫
5. 炒至開始變焦黃
6. 加入雞蛋
7. 把雞蛋炒散，讓雞蛋和姜融合一起
8. 轉小火
9. 把剩米飯倒入並炒散
10. 加入適量的鹽
11. 把米飯攤平在底內，讓火慢慢的米飯烘得干

Ginger Fried Rice

1 bowl of day-old rice

2 eggs

1 piece of ginger

pinch of salt

1. Peel ginger (skin may be left on for better nutrition)

2. Julienne ginger.

3. Add oil onto a heated pan.

4. Add ginger and cook until golden.

6. Add and scramble eggs with ginger.

8. Reduce to low heat.

9. Add rice and stir fry it.

10. Add salt.

11. Spread the rice to the bottom of the pan and cook at low heat to allow moisture to evaporate.

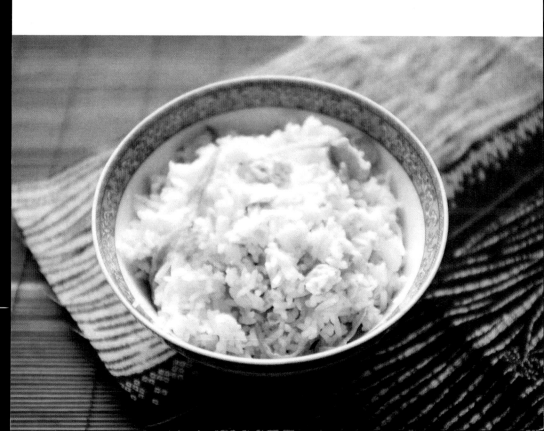

豬脚黑米醋

黑米醋 1 樽~ 600mL 或更多,
如果需要添加

豬手 (或豬脚) 2-3 隻 可以剁
成中或小塊

糖 1 tsp 或更多,如果需要添
加

水或雞湯 1 c

雞蛋 2-4隻 或更多

大塊薑 ~1 lb. 或多或少-按照
自己的喜好

1.洗淨豬脚/手,用鹽洗皮，清掉豬毛

2.把豬脚/手在熱水裡滾一滾.

3.把豬脚/手在凍水裡,然後出水

4.用另外一個煲 煮雞蛋,大約12分鐘

5.拿出來,放在凍水裡,會容易剝蛋殼

6.洗薑塊,可以輕輕拍扁薑

7.炒一炒薑

8.加入黑米醋,少量糖(帶有酸甜味就可
以) 大約15 分鐘 (如果太酸，可依據自
己的喜好加水或雞湯來調節口味)

9.加入豬脚/手 , 蛋

10.讓它煮到豬脚/手軟了(用一根筷子戳
如果你喜歡軟一點,可以繼續煮*

Pig Trotters in
Ginger and Sweetened Vinegar

600mL of black rice vinegar

2-3 pieces of pig trotters

1 tablespoon of sugar

1 cup water or chicken broth

2-4 eggs

1 lb large ginger pieces

1. Wash pig trotters first, and then rub skin with salt, remove hair if necessary.

2. Quickly cook in boiling water and remove.

3. Place trotters in cold water, then drain.

4. Boil eggs in a separate pot for about 12 minutes.

5. Remove from heat and place in cold water to more easily peel eggshell.

6. Wash ginger and lightly pound ginger.

7. Stir fry ginger in a pot for a few minutes.

8. Add black rice vinegar and some sugar to reach a sweet-and-sour taste. Cook for about 15 minutes (adjust taste with water or chicken broth).

9. Add pig trotters and eggs to the pot.

10. Let it cook until pig trotters are soft (test by poking with a chopstick). Boil longer if you prefer tender meat.

红糖煮荷包蛋

水

红糖

鸡蛋

配伍

加入当归、山药、党参、薏仁、枸杞、红枣一起炖，有利于身体恢复

1.首先水烧开（一碗水）

2.然後加入大約兩勺紅糖（根據個人口味，若喜歡甜味可多加點）

3.再把鸡蛋打开放进去，中火煮五分钟（喜歡較老的口感的可煮七八分鐘）

Boiled Egg in Brown Sugar

water

brown sugar

eggs

Optional:
Angelica, yam, Codonopsis,
barley, wolfberry, red dates

1. First boil a bowl of water, then add two spoonfuls of brown sugar (adjust to taste).

2. Beat the eggs in a bowl and add to boiling water.

3. Simmer over medium heat for five minutes (or seven to eight minutes if you prefer firmer texture).

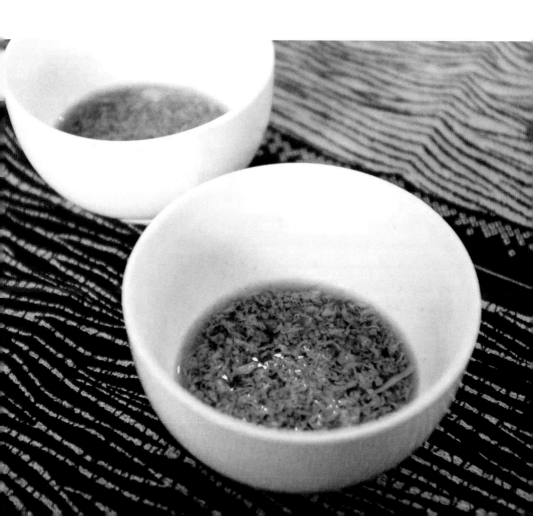

THANK YOU

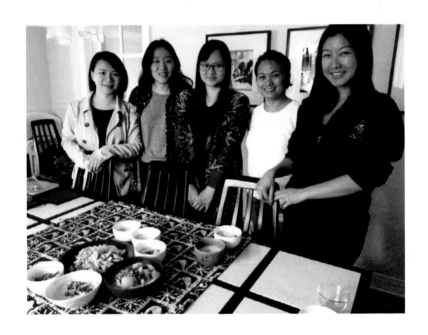

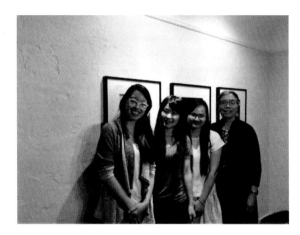

Natalie Hsueh (left),
Candas Tsai, Khanh-Hoa
Nguyen, Dr. Marilyn Wong
(right)

Kim Thuy Ho
Leigh Ann Llarena
Stephanie Yom
Fay Pon
Khanh-Hoa Nguyen
Dr. Marilyn Wong

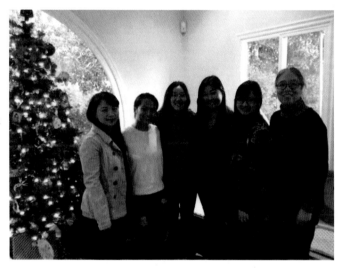

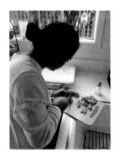
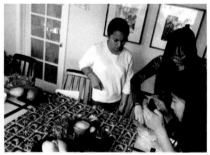
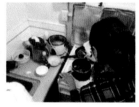